UNDERSTANDING SUICIDE

By Patricia Carlisle

TABLE OF CONTENT

Introduction

I want to thank you and congratulate you for choosing the book, *"UNDERSTANDING SUICIDE."*

This book contains the framework to understanding suicide, methods on suicide prevention, and causes of suicide.

Suicide is not a new phenomenon. Strikingly, accounts of suicide across the last millennium catalogue the same factors associated with suicide as those revealed by modern scientific study in western cultures; serious mental illness, alcohol and substance abuse, co-morbidity, childhood abuse, loss of a love one, fear of humiliation, and economic dislocation, and insecurity.

Thanks again for downloading this book, I hope you enjoy it!

Chapter 1

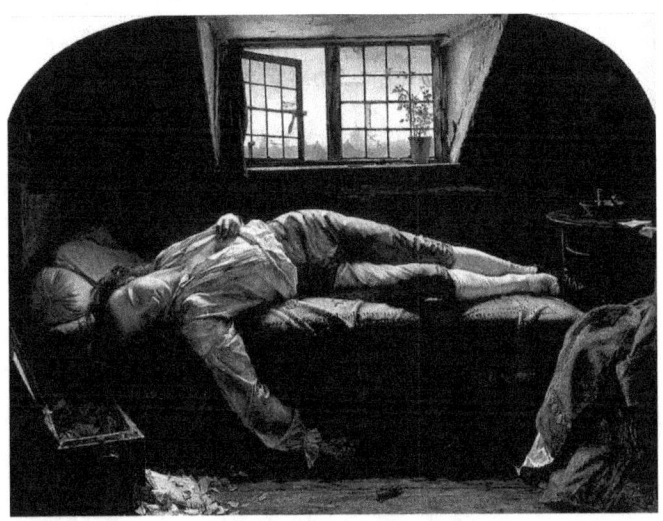

SUICIDE THROUGH HISTORY

Every year approximately 30,000 people die by suicide in
United States, and one million worldwide. Approximately
650,000 people yearly receive emergency treatment after
attempting suicide in United States. It is the third leading
course of death among American youths, and the eleventh for
Americans of all ages. Over the last 100 years suicides have
out-numbered homicides by at least 3 to 2. Almost 4 times as
many Americans died by suicide than in the Vietnam War
during this same time period.

The rates of suicide are exceptionally high among certain
populations; white males over 75 years of age, Native
Americans, and certain profession (e.g., health professions,
police). The rates among youth are rising. For decades, the
federal government of the United States has been concerned
about high suicide rates. Thirty years after the first national
effort was established at the National Institute of Mental

Health in 1969, the Surgeon General of the United States issued a "Call to Action to Prevent Suicide." Soon after, a National Strategy for Suicide Prevention (2001), presented a comprehensive assessment of future goals and objectives to combat suicide.

Several federal agencies (the National Institute of Mental Health, the National Institute of Drug Abuse, the Veterans Administration, the Centers for Disease control and Prevention, Substance Abuse and Mental Health Services Administration, and the National Institute on Alcohol Abuse and Alcoholism); joined together to ask the Institute of Medicine to convene the committee on Pathophysiology and Prevention of Adolescent and Adult Suicide to examine the state of the science base, gaps in our knowledge, strategies for prevention, and research designs for the study of suicide.

Chapter 2

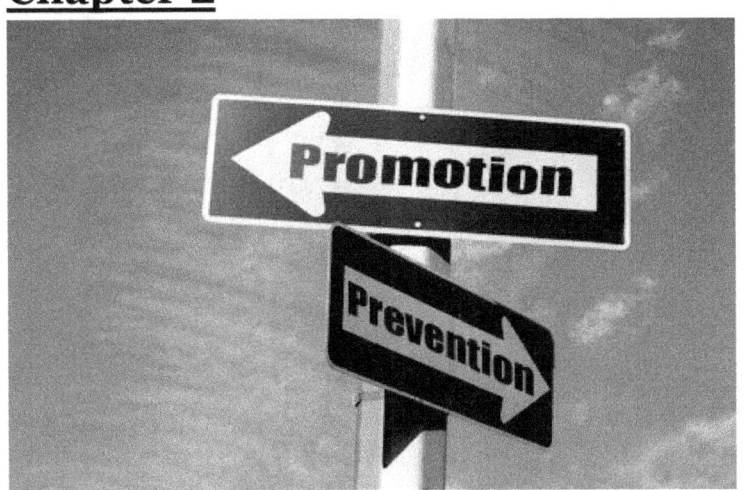

FRAMEWORK FOR PREVENTION
Universal Selective and Indicated Prevention Model:

The prevailing prevention model in the interdisciplinary field of prevention science is the Universal Selective, and Indicated (USI) prevention model. This USI model focuses attention on defined populations-from everyone in the population, to specific at-risk groups, to specific high-risk individuals-i.e., three population groups for whom the designed interventions are deemed optimal for achieving the unique goals of each prevention type.

Prevention Programs

Universal strategies, or initiatives address an entire population (the nation, state, Local County or community, school or neighborhood). These prevention programs are designed to influence everyone, reducing suicide risk though removing barriers to care, enhancing knowledge of what to do and say to help suicidal individuals, increasing access to help, and strengthening protective process like social support and coping skills.

Universal interventions include programs such as public education campaigns, school-based "suicide awareness" programs, means restriction, education programs for the media on reporting practices related to suicide, and school-based crisis response plans and teams.

Selective strategies address subsets of the total population, focusing on at-risk groups that have a greater probability of becoming suicidal. Selective prevention strategies aim to prevent the onset of suicidal behaviors among specific subpopulations. This level of prevention include programs, gatekeeper training for "frontline" adult caregivers, and peer "natural helpers," support and skill building groups for at-risk groups in the population, and enhanced accessible crisis services, and referral sources. **Indicated strategies** address specific high-risk individuals within the population-those evidencing early signs of suicide potential. **Programs** are designed and delivered in groups or individually to reduce risk factors, and increase protective factors. At this level, **programs include** skill building support groups in high schools and colleges, parent support training programs, case management for individual high-risk youth at school, and referral sources for crisis intervention and treatment.

Chapter 3

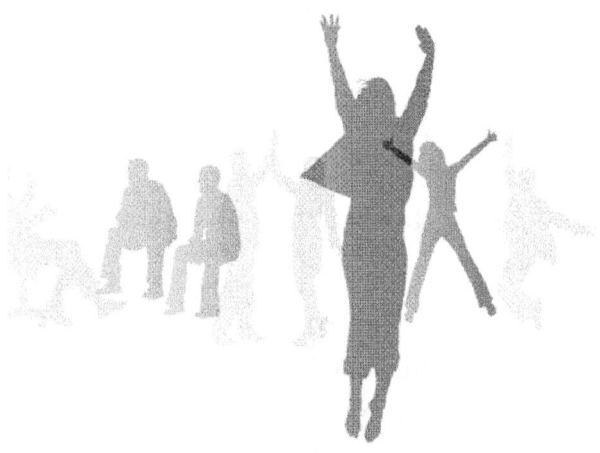

UNIVERSAL PREVENTIONS
Health Promotion Strategies

Using health promotion strategies to combat symptoms of mental illness, including suicidality, represent a primary aspect of many universal suicide prevention programs. Although the field has traditionally separated health promotion from prevention (IOM, 1944), research shows, prevention experts in the United States and abroad have increasingly turned to mental health promotion as a means of universal prevention. At least one expert in meta-analysis demonstrate that school-based programs employing such a health promotion approach can effectively prevent, and/or reduce suicide risk factors, and correlates like adolescent pregnancy, externalizing disorders (such as delinquency and substance abuse), and depression.

These programs also promote protective factors against suicide including: self-efficacy, interpersonal problem solving, self esteem, and social. Furthermore, throughout the 1990s, the World Health Organization developed evidence-based policies, and recommendations for how schools can effectively engage in health promotion using a four level model (see, WHO, 2002). The **WHO model** promotes universal prevention, targeting environmental conditions and mental health education for all students, as well as selective and indicated prevention, providing psychosocial interventions, and professional treatment for those with mental illness, or at significant risk says experts.

The U.S. Surgeon General, the United Nations, and the World Health Organization have endorsed promoting mental health/resiliency as part of universal suicide reduction strategies. Population-based prevention programs with a school or community focus have an important advantage over those aimed at individuals. There is usually a high participation rate in such programs because all students are exposed, for instance, to a teacher's classroom management practices, and control of aggressive behavior, or to a middle school drug prevention program.

These programs also have the advantage because of inoculation, of having potential impact on not only those who are currently at risk, but also those whose risk status changes after the intervention takes place. Finally, many of these broad prevention programs target multiple outcomes, so overall risk for suicide may be reduced by diminishing developmental risk through multiple pathways. **Policy changes** represent another universal strategy for reducing suicide. For example, experts conclude in a review of minimum drinking age policies in each state from 1970 to 1990 that increase in the legal drinking age reduce not only motor vehicle deaths, but also suicides.

Chapter 4

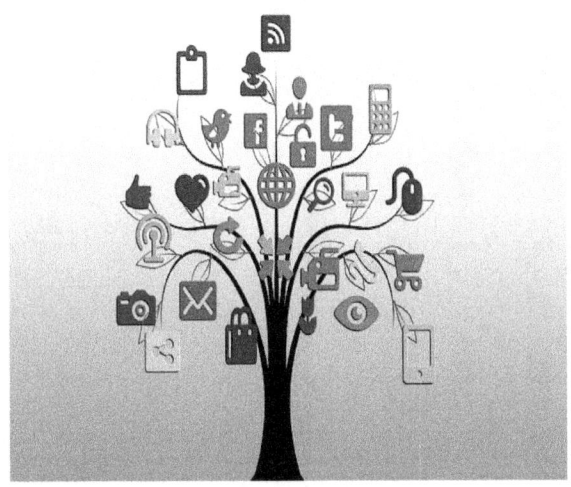

MEDIA CAMPAIGNS
Universal Public Health approach

A traditional universal public health approach to behavior-related problems has been widespread education through mass-media campaigns. According to research, this technique has been used with varying levels of success for smoking, AIDS, and coronary heart disease.

A few countries, including the United Kingdom and Norway, have implemented such mass-media campaigns for suicide prevention as part of overall mental health promotion; evaluations of results are not yet available. Extensive media campaigns for suicide prevention are not common, largely due to fear of engendering suicide imitation.

Media initiatives more often have focused on modifying portrayals of suicide to reduce the likelihood of imitation. Since data are limited on use of media for education, Next, I will discuss what is known about suicide imitation through the media, followed by a description of efforts to address this problem, and the evidence for their effectiveness.

Chapter 5

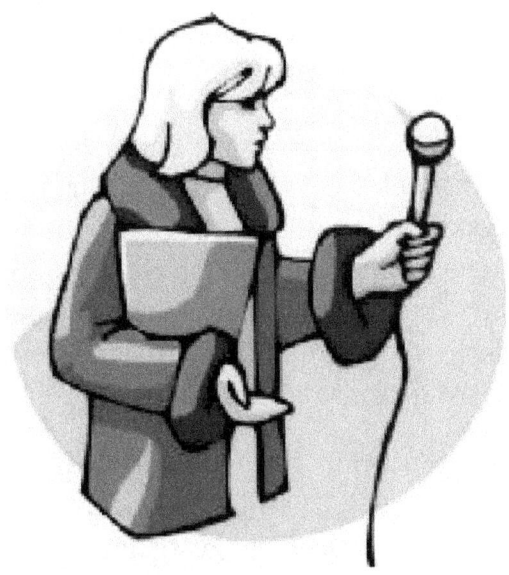

IMITATION THROUGH THE MEDIA

Throughout history, people have expressed concern about suicide imitation, and have seen the opportunity for intervention in such matters, as evidenced by various unreliable accounts in the literature of suicide imitation and clustering. For example, Goethe's 1773 novel, The Sorrows of Young Werther, in which the title character shoots himself after a failed love affair, was banned in Denmark, Saxony, and Milan in order to prevent further suicides that were thoughts to be a result of young men imitating the behavior of Werther (Phillips, 1974,1985). These events led to the term "Werther Effect" being used to describe imitation of this sort. Today this effect is referred to as either suicide contagion or suicide imitation/modeling.

Although they are often used interchangeably, each is based on a different theoretical framework. Each theoretical framework is useful, but some experts propose that the language of imitation and modeling is preferable to the language of a contagious process; because it relies on active learning processes that do not imply the exclusion of individual volitional factors.

Imitation and modeling, which play a role in other harmful behaviors such as drug use and bullying, occur with suicide in several circumstances, such as in the case of temporal clusters of suicides in a particular community or culture, suicide among family members, and suicide following exposure to a medial presentation of a real of fictional suicide.

Research shows that suicide contagion through the media is real. Recent meta-analyses report that studies conducted by clinically oriented investigators yield the strongest support for suicide imitation. However, many of the studies of suicide imitation are beset with methodological problems; for example, many are based on aggregate level data, which preclude the possibility of ruling out the influence of other factors.

Imitation can be linked to newspaper accounts of suicide. Newspaper coverage of suicide is related to an increase in the rate of suicide, and the magnitude of the increase is proportional to the duration, prominence and amount of media coverage. There has been less conclusive research on the consequences of television news programs on suicide imitation. Experts found no association over an 11 year period in the United States, but recent studies suggest imitation in specific groups. The influence of fictional presentations of suicide on imitation is less clear.

Research into fictional portrayals has examined attempts, or other suicidal behavior (such as ideation) rather than just rates of completed suicides, which allows for actual measurement of exposure.   Some studies indicate that imitation occurs. Aspects of both the media presentation, and the individual interact to produce imitation. This person is likely to imitate a suicidal behavior.

Media Intimidation

Media refers to literature, the press, music, broadcasting, films, TV, theater, and the Internet has underlying vulnerabilities. A healthy person is not likely to kill him or herself as a result of seeing an example of suicide. Different media (e.g., book vs. television) are likely to exert differential effects on different populations. Both the form of headline, placement, and content (celebrity, mental illness, and murder-suicide) of suicide coverage clearly impact the likelihood of imitation.

Attractive models are more likely to cause imitation. Similarities between a vulnerable person, and the reported suicide victim increase the likelihood of contagion. This has been shown with age effects in both the young and the elderly. Similarly, ethnicity is an important factor; experts found that suicides of foreigners did not cause imitation among native populations.

Chapter 6

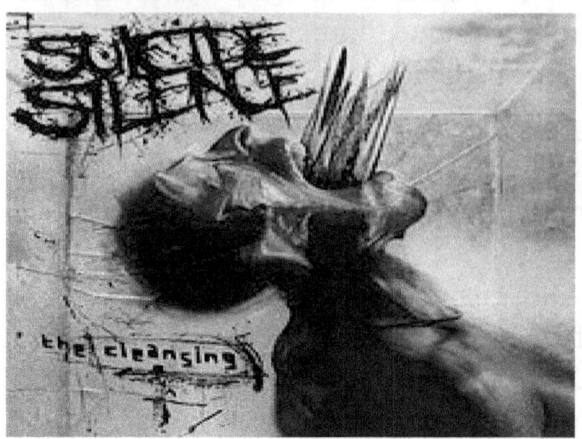

ENCOURAGING RESPONSIBLE ON COVERAGE SUICIDE

Many elements of media presentations influence the likelihood of imitation, and these all provide opportunities for prevention. In efforts to prevent contagion, several countries (including Australia, Austria, Canada, Germany, Japan, New Zealand, and Switzerland), and organizations; including the World Health Organization (United Nations, 1996; WHO, 2000b) have formulated guidelines for media coverage of suicide. The National Strategy for Suicide Prevention in the United States as one of its major goals improving "the reporting and portrayals of suicidal behavior, mental illness, and substance abuse in the entertainment, and news media."

To advance that goal, guidelines for media coverage of suicide were formulated by the Annenberg Public Policy Center of the University of Pennsylvania, the American Association of Suicidology (AAS), and the American Foundation for Suicide Prevention (AFSP) in collaboration with several government agencies (CDC, NIMH, Office of the Surgeon General,

Substance Abuse and Mental health Services Administration SAMSHA), the WHO, and other international suicide prevention groups.

They were released in August 2001, and the full text of these guidelines can be found on the sites of the partner organizations that developed them, including www.appcpenn.org, and www.afsp.org. These guidelines, "Reporting on Suicide: Recommendations for the Media" update those developed in 1989 at a national consensus conference on the topic.

The media guidelines include the stipulation that media accounts of suicide should neither romanticize nor normalize suicide; that is, individuals who kill themselves should not inadvertently be idealized a heroic or romantic. They also urge the inclusion of factual information on suicide contagion and mental illness, provide suggestions for questions to ask of relatives and friends of the victim, and suggest that information on treatment resources be included.

The guidelines also address issues of language such as the use of terms like "a successful suicide," and speak to special situations that may arise such as a celebrity death by suicide. Finally, they suggest that media professionals address suicide as an issue in its own right, reporting on stigma, treatments, and trends I suicide rates, rather than only in response to a tragedy.

With shifts in focus and inclusion of educational material, the same articles that report on an unfortunate event can become part of universal preventive measures.

The echoes other areas in the injury prevention field; the media now indicate the status of smoke detectors when a fire is reported, for example. Likewise, helmet use is indicated when reporting a bicycle incident. Currently, many comprehensive suicide prevention programs include components to improve media response to suicide, including the Finland National Program, Maryland and the Washington State Youth Suicide Prevention Program, and a state programs often utilizing the nationally formulated guidelines. The Washington program included a media education component that was designed to impact reporting practices by:

- Educating media personnel in ways to report youth suicide stories that prevent potential contagion effects

- and Educating select personnel such as crisis line workers, gatekeepers, and school personnel in how to respond to media requests for information and stories related to youth suicide and suicide prevention. It also focused on ensuring that the youth suicide prevention message was "in the news" by providing information to the media, and encouraging ongoing and responsible coverage of suicide, and suicide prevention/reduced thoughts.

Despite such efforts to shape discussion of suicide in the media, very little evidence exist to show the initiatives to promote responsible reporting in the media have a direct significant effect on suicide rates. In Switzerland, implementation of media guidelines did increase responsible reporting of suicides; less sensational, and higher quality stories resulted.

But this has not yet been related to changes in suicide rates. An evaluation of media guidelines in Austria showed significant success in reducing suicides. The guidelines in the country were specifically formulated to address concerns that the increase in the number of suicides, and suicide attempts on the subway in Vienna was related to the highly publicized, and dramatic accounts of the deaths.

Subsequent to the release of the guidelines, newspaper reporting of subway suicides decreased greatly, and what was reported was much less prominent. The number of subway suicides significantly decreased in the second half of the year after release. In the 4 years following, the overall suicide rate decreased by 20 percent, and the rate of subway suicides decreased by 75 percent with no substitution of method.

Chapter 7

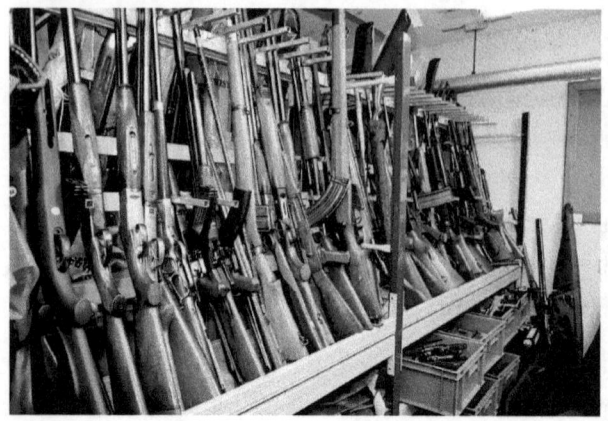

REDUCING ACCESS TO MEANS

Universal measures can be used to reduce the availability of common tools for suicide. More restrictive legislation regarding firearms, barriers on bridges, or blister packs for medications are interventions that may be effective in reducing suicide, or suicide attempts. This section focuses on the role of availability of methods of suicide, including the role that method availability and barrier restrictions may play in suicide by firearms, overdose, prescription drugs, jumping from buildings or bridges, domestic gas, automobile carbon monoxide, and railway suicides. Much of the research discussed has been done in Western societies, but suicide in rural Asian societies has been largely linked with availability of insecticides. Research is limited, but this underscores the need for implementing safe storage of agricultural poisons, and using safety caps to reduce impulsive swallowing.

Firearms

Epidemiological studies have consistently shown that firearms are most common method of suicide for all demographic groups in the United States. The association between suicide and firearms in the home is strong access among all age groups, but is particularly high in the 24 and younger group of 10.4 vs. 4.0-7.2 for those 25 and older). The dramatic increase in the American youth suicide rate since 1960 is primarily attributable to an increase in suicide by firearms. In one study of youth suicide in Allegheny County form 1960-1983, the rate of suicide by firearms increased 330 percent, but the rate of suicide by other means increased only 150 percent. The more recent increase in the suicide rate by African American males is also attributable primarily to an increase in suicide by firearms. The Odds Ratio is the ratio of the odds of an outcome (suicide) for the experimental group relative to the odds of the outcome in the control group.

Chapter 8

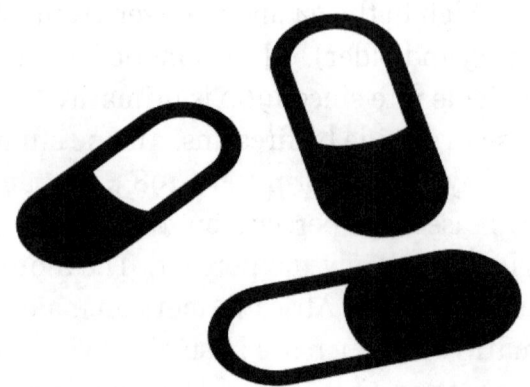

ACETAMINOPHEN OVERDOSE

The rate of acetaminophen (or paracetamol) self-poisoning from emergency room registries has been estimated 21.4 per 100,000 in one American emergency room, and as high as 70-90 per 1000,0000 in one study based in Scotland. In the Scottish study, the rates among male and female adolescents aged 15-19 were approximate 150 and 350 per 100,000, respectively. Hospitalizations due to acetaminophen rose rapidly from the 1970s through the early 1990s especially in adolescents and young adults. This increase is explained in part by the increased availability of acetaminophen.

High correlations have been noted between sales of acetaminophen and overdose rates in Oxford, England (r=.86), and in France (r=.99), with similar correlations between sales and completed suicide. In addition to availability, adolescents' general ignorance about the risk for hepatotoxicity appears to contribute to the use of acetaminophen. Almost half of adolescents underestimate the potential lethality and toxicity of acetaminophen.

Awareness is also limited that ingestion of acetaminophen in combination with alcohol greatly increases the likelihood of both hospitalization and hepatotoxicity. Restriction of drug content per purchase, and the use of blister packs (requiring individual pill removal from a card with each pill in its own "bubble" may reduce the morbidity and mortality due to acetaminophen overdose). Restriction in the amount of drug available in a purchase resulted in a 4-fold lower fatality from overdose in France, compared to England.

The introduction of blister packs as a method for dispensing acetaminophen was associated with a 21 percent reduction in overdoses and a 64-percent reduction in severe overdoses, whereas overdoses due to benzodiazepines, which were not subject to these restrictions, remained stable. Some have considered the benefit of labels warning of hepatotoxicity, but it is unclear if warnings would alter the behavior of impulsive adolescents.

In addition of methionine to prevent the hepatotoxic effects has been suggested but not yet evaluated. Therefore, to reduce suicide thoughts, acetaminophen overdose injection must be kept far away from people.

Chapter 9

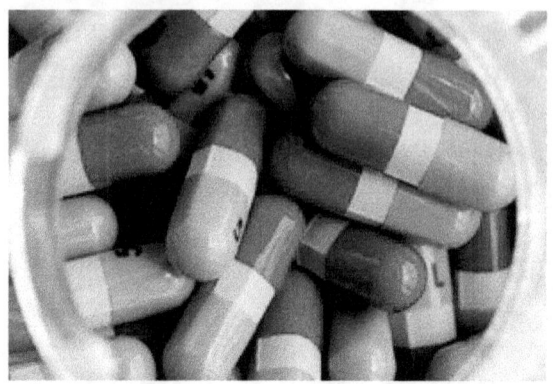

PRESCRIPTION DRUGS

Research shows, the rate of self-poisoning by prescription drugs in New York City is highest in Manhattan, which has the higher per-capita density of physicians of any of the boroughs of New York. The greater number of prescribed psychotropic agents is correlated with an increased risk of overdose, at an estimated rate of 3.8 per 1000 prescriptions. However, researchers found no relationship between availability of prescription drugs, and complete suicide. The prescription of a psychotropic agent is itself a marker for suicidal risk, and it is important to consider its lethality in prescribing for patients with mental disorders. Furthermore, there is a marked gradient in toxicity among antidepressants.

In a study conducted in the United Kingdom, desipramine was reported to have over twice the death rate by overdose per 1,000,000 prescriptions compared to amitriptyline, imipramine, or nortriptyline, and 9 times the death rate by overdose of mianserin.

In data from the United States, the toxicity of different antidepressants was examined using two different databases, the Association of Poison Control Centers (APCC), and the Drug Abuse and Early Warning Network (DAWN). In the APCC database the rate of overdose was adjusted for prescription volume based on the National Prescription Audit. Both APCC and DAWN databases revealed that desipramine had a higher risk for suicide attempt, and greater fatality given an overdose than either amiriptyline or imipramine. The DAWN analysis also demonstrated that the three tricyclic antidepressants had between a 2.5 and 8.5 greater risk of death due to overdose than fluoxetine.

Therefore, alteration in prescription practices to favor SSRIs over TCAs might result in a decline in deaths by overdose of antidepressants. Experts believe suicide and suicide attempt are markedly increased in patients with epilepsy.

While interictal psychopathology related to epilepsy seems to be an important risk factor for suicidal behavior, Phenobarbital may be an iatrogenic cause of depression, and suicidal behavior in epilepsy. One naturalistic study suggested that exposure to Phenobarbital caused about a 4-fold risk for depression, which was most likely to occur if there was a family history of depression, and very unlikely to occur in the absence of a family history of depression. Phenobarbital is no longer a first-line anticonvulsant in the United States, but because of its overall safety and cost, it still is used quite commonly in developing countries. Screening for a family history of depression may help to avoid the iatrogenic difficulties associated with this medication, and reduce suicide thought and feelings.

Chapter 10

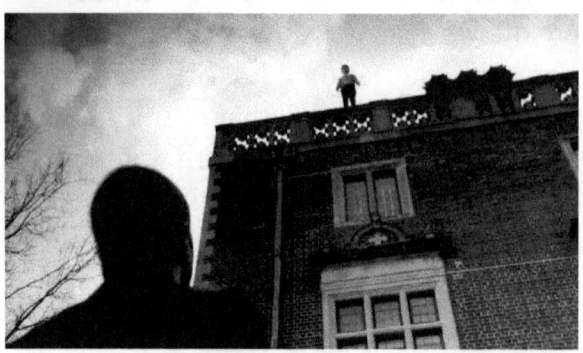

JUMPING FROM BUILDINGS OR BRIDGES

Availability of high buildings or bridges provides another means for suicide. In New York City, suicide by jumping was highest in Manhattan, and lowest in Staten Island, the two extremes fro access to building of 7 stories or higher.

In another study in new York, 81 percent of all suicides jumped from their own residences. One report suggested the efficacy of crisis telephone line on a bridge. Its use in 30 cases result cases resulted in only one completed suicide.

Nine people jumped from the bridge, and did not use the phone; 5 of the 9 completed the suicide. The availability of the phone line, staffed by mental health experts, and with an automatic police alert, may have deterred some suicides.

As with injury control approaches, the creation of mechanical barriers on bridges could make jumping more difficult, or impossible. Mechanical barriers in private residences would be more difficult to develop and enforce.

Chapter 11

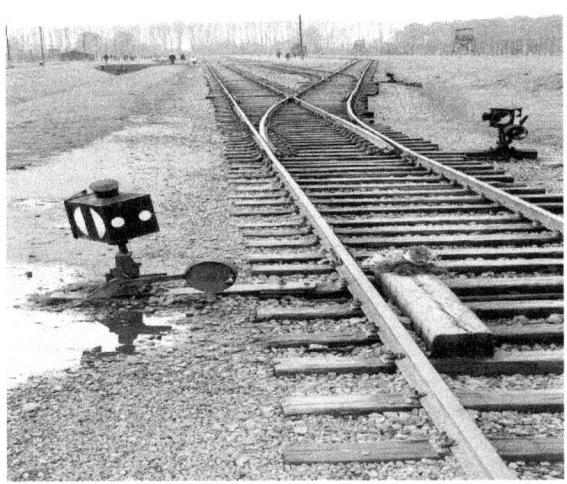

DOMESTIC GAS POISONING/RAILWAY SUICIDES

Domestic gas poisoning was one of the leading causes of suicide of Great Britain; due to its high carbon monoxide (CO) content, domestic gas could be highly lethal. A decrease in CO content of domestic gas associated with decline in mortality in Great Britain, Austria, and Japan, but not in the Netherlands.

Method substitution eventually offset the decline in suicide by the mid-1980s in Great Britain, but not Japan. Therefore, in some locales, the detoxification of domestic gas has had a lasting effect, and even in Great Britain, where method substitution did eventually take place, this occurred after a reduction in the suicide rate which lasted for a 15-year period.

Railway Suicides

The rate of railway suicide (e.g., jumping in front of a train) also is related to access. In New York, the rate of railway or subway suicide is proportional to the amount of track in a given borough. However, among cities internationally, there are marked variations in the suicide rate per passenger. Rates are extremely low in Singapore, Tokyo, Budapest, and Hong Kong, but much higher in London, Barcelona, Rio de Janeiro, and Paris.

Because the case fatality rate is high (estimated at 55 percent) and prediction is difficult, injury control methods have been suggest to reduce fatality. Suggestions include physical separation of passengers for the train bed, improved surveillance of passengers by station staff, liaison to hospital staff in stations with a high density of chronic mental patients, availability of emergency hotline telephones, redesign of bumper of train (including the addition of an airbag), increasing the distance between the train and the train bed, and a slower speed of approach to the station.

In addition to design issues, curbing media publicity about railway suicides may diminish the likelihood of imitation.

Conclusion

Thank you again for choosing this book!

I hope this book was able to help you understand Suicide and suicide prevention.

The next step is to look-up some of the programs that's mentioned throughout this book and share them with others in need.

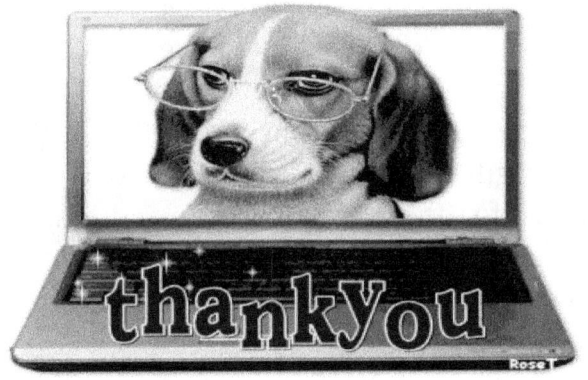

Finally, if you enjoyed this book would you be kind enough to leave a review for this book on Amazon? It'd be greatly appreciated!

Leave a review for this book on Amazon.com!

Thank you and good luck!

Preview Of 'THOUGHT WITHOUT THINKING: Taking control over your racing thoughts'

Chapter 1
RACING THOUGHTS

Racing thoughts are a strange issue. It's not simply the substance of the idea. It's the way it feels as if your thoughts are firing at such a quick pace, to the point that you can't considerably recall what the last thought was, and when you have another thought another instantly takes its place. Racing thoughts may influence anybody with anxiety; however it is most common for those that have anxiety attacks. Racing thoughts might likewise influence those with summed up anxiety issue, and may influence about anybody with an issue when they encounter serious anxiety.

It's likewise extremely common at sleep. For reasons unknown, numerous individuals discover that their thoughts appear to be quicker when they're attempting to get to sleep, and shockingly when they happen amid bed time it can be difficult to get any sleep. The reasons for racing thoughts are likely identified with the way your neurotransmitters interface aid anxiety, alongside the surge of adrenaline you get when you have anxiety (which may make your mind significantly more dynamic). Adrenaline, particularly, causes your psyche to be over-dynamic while at the same time making it harder to core interest. Different reasons may include: One of the reasons they happen when you're attempting to go to rest is on account of there are no diversions. When you're left with your own thoughts, your thoughts regularly go unchecked, and in the end they winding wild.

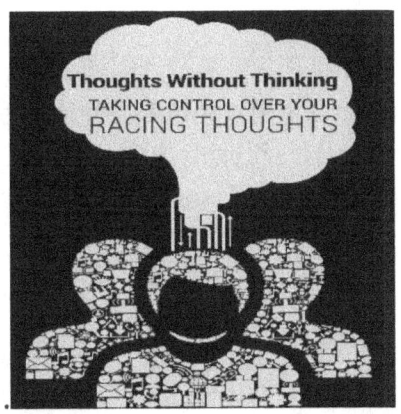

 To check out the rest of (THOUGHT WITHOUT THINKING: Taking control over your racing thoughts) on Amazon.

Check Out My Other Books

Below you'll find some of my other popular books that are popular on Amazon and Kindle as well. Simply click on the links below to check them out. Alternatively, you can visit my author page on Amazon to see other work done by me.

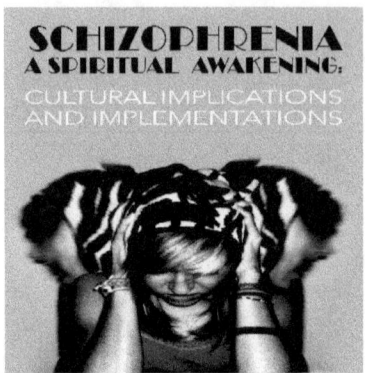

Schizophrenia a spiritual awakening: Cultural implications and implementations.

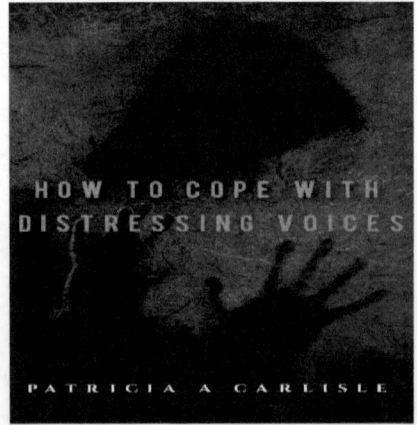

How to cope with distressing voices.

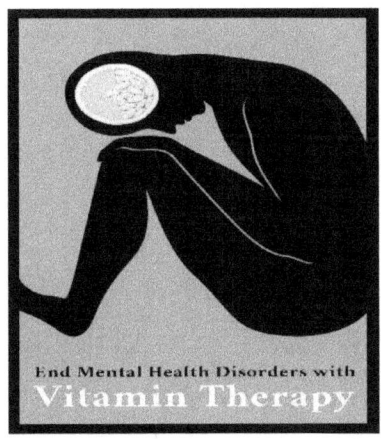

End Mental Disorders with vitamin therapy. Download here:

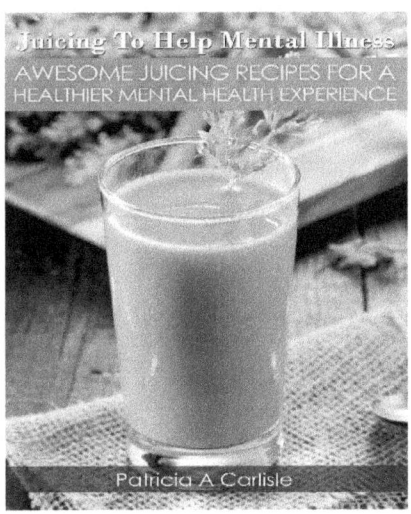

Juicing to Help Mental Illness: Awesome juicing recipes for a healthier mental health.

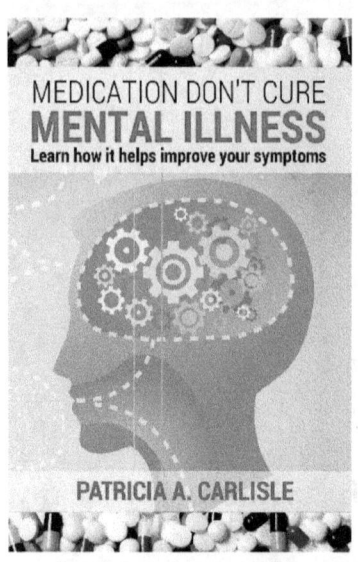

MEDICATION DON'T CURE MENTAL ILLNESS: Learn how it helps improve your symptoms.

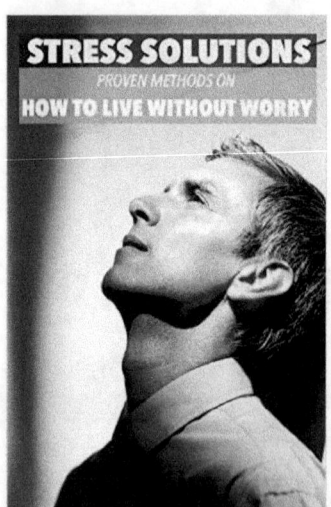

STRESS SOLUTIONS: Proven methods on how to live without worry.

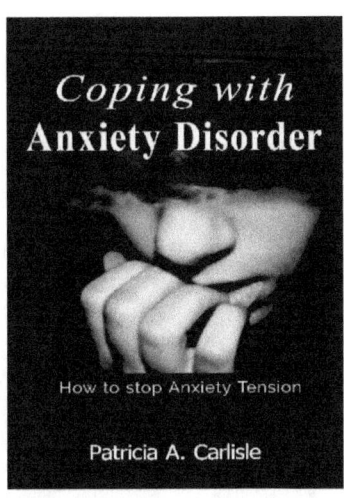

Coping with Anxiety Disorder: How to stop Anxiety Tension. Download here:

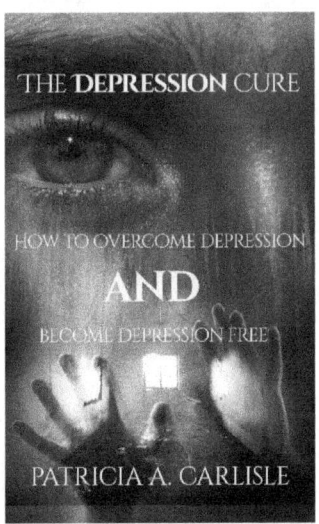

THE DEPRESSION CURE: How to overcome depression and become depression free.

NOTE

NOTES

NOTES

www.ingramcontent.com/pod-product-compliance
Lightning Source LLC
Chambersburg PA
CBHW071019180526
45168CB00003B/1487